MW00975156

Freedom
from
Fibromyalgia Pain

REV. KATHY VENS

WESTBOW
PRESS
A DIVISION OF THOMAS NELSON

Copyright © 2013 Rev. Kathy Vens.

All rights reserved. No part of this book may be used or reproduced by any means, graphic, electronic, or mechanical, including photocopying, recording, taping or by any information storage retrieval system without the written permission of the publisher except in the case of brief quotations embodied in critical articles and reviews.

All biblical references are taken from the New King James Version and King James Version of the Bible.

Scripture taken from the New King James Version. Copyright 1979, 1980, 1982 by Thomas Nelson, inc. Used by permission. All rights reserved.

Scripture taken from the King James Version of the Bible.

WestBow Press books may be ordered through booksellers or by contacting:

WestBow Press
A Division of Thomas Nelson
1663 Liberty Drive
Bloomington, IN 47403
www.westbowpress.com
1-(866) 928-1240

Because of the dynamic nature of the Internet, any web addresses or links contained in this book may have changed since publication and may no longer be valid. The views expressed in this work are solely those of the author and do not necessarily reflect the views of the publisher, and the publisher hereby disclaims any responsibility for them.

Any people depicted in stock imagery provided by Thinkstock are models, and such images are being used for illustrative purposes only.

Certain stock imagery © Thinkstock.

ISBN: 978-1-4497-9418-7 (sc)
ISBN: 978-1-4497-9420-0 (e)
Library of Congress Control Number: 2013908039
Printed in the United States of America.

WestBow Press rev. date: 5/6/2013

Contents

If you live according to the flesh you will die;

but if by the Spirit you put to death

the deeds of the body, you will live.

For as many as are led by the Spirit of God,

these are the sons of God.

Romans 8:13-14 (NKJV)

This book is dedicated with humble gratitude to Jesus Christ who loves me and gave me the strength and power to write this book. He deserves all glory for His wonderful work in me.

To my sons, Zachary and Colton: thank you for all the years you dealt with my going through so much pain and not understanding the reason why I couldn't get well. I love you both dearly and hope this explanation will help you through life. You have both taught me so much through your own lifestyles of eating healthfully and from the land. God bless you both in your life adventures and your health.

I also dedicate this book to those who are fighting fibromyalgia and diseases that cause excruciating pain. I hope and pray this book will lead you to the One who brings healing to us through different avenues.

1

Direction in My Life

Have you ever felt you were supposed to do something, but you just didn't know what that something was? That feeling has been with me for a few years now, and I've concluded that the Holy Spirit has been nudging me to write a book. I kept putting it off—I often thought of things I could write about, but nothing really stuck. So I asked, "Lord, what am I supposed to write about that other people have not already covered a few hundred times?" The one thing that kept coming to my mind and spirit was my diagnosis of fibromyalgia.

I knew that Psalm 146:7 says, *"…The Lord gives freedom to the prisoners."* I believe that God gives freedom to each of us, and that will happen either on this side of heaven or when we get there and are face-to-face with our Savior. Our God is a healer and deliverer. He came to set the captives free! Nothing is impossible with God.

No matter if it's a food addiction, alcohol, drugs, pain, tobacco, or a sexual addiction, gossip, fear, unbelief, or unforgiveness I believe our God can free us from the shackles of sin.

Jesus is the light of the world and in Him there is no darkness. First John 1:5 says, "*...God is light and in Him is no darkness at all.*" Every time light comes to the darkness in our life the darkness must flee. Light dispels the darkness. Truth and knowledge will give you strength to stand against the enemy of your soul. The more of God's Word that is in you the more you can be bold and courageous and not be terrified or discouraged because our Lord is with us wherever we go and whatever we do. (Joshua 1:9)

Let the peace of God shine forth in you as you read this book and let His truth be in you. He is the One who gives us His Holy Spirit to guide us into all truth.

2

Living with Fibromyalgia Pain

Pain is either acute or chronic. Acute pain is normal pain that lets you know that you've been hurt—for example, when you hit your finger with a hammer or break a leg. Chronic pain is ongoing lasting for weeks, months, or even years—far beyond the time of expected recovery. Fibromyalgia pain is usually chronic, and as of this writing, there is no cure. Pain interacts with our emotions as it moves and interacts through the body. Pain then seems to affect our spirit.

When we are in pain spiritually, the body works hand in hand with our spirit. To mingle the physical life with the mental and spiritual comes naturally, because we live in the image of God, and He is triune. He is the Father, Son, and Holy Spirit. Jesus was made flesh to know our pain and feel it. The Holy Spirit knows our innermost thoughts and desires as God, the Father created us.

Our physical life has a definite effect on our spiritual life. I'm a living example of the physical, emotional and spiritual coming together and working itself out within me. At age fifteen, I was a blonde, green-eyed young lady who had been raised to look at work as something fun to do. It seemed logical, as working was how my family spent a good portion of our lives. I figured if I went to work at a job away from home, I would at least be paid for doing something, and then I wouldn't have to work as hard at home.

I worked very hard in a restaurant. I waited on tables, cooked, scrubbed floors, cleaned the walk-in cooler, ice-cream maker, and washed many dishes (the restaurant didn't have a dishwasher back then). I also did payroll, which kept me very busy at times.

My brother worked with me, and we would compete all the time to see which of us could do things faster. One of those things was cutting up boxes of chickens. We would put the chickens on the chopping blocks and go at it, timing each other to see who was faster at cutting up those chickens. We found joy in almost anything that was good, clean fun. We really enjoyed working together.

As I look back now, I still remember how much pain I was in, almost daily. I often thought, *If I feel this bad now, how will I feel at age forty?* Forty years of age seemed old back then to me. It seems just a few years ago, although I am now pushing fifty-three years of age.

In my twenties, life was very stressful. I went through several challenges and truly believe God carried me the whole way—I wouldn't be here today if it was not for the grace of God. I lived in a tormented relationship with a man who verbally, sexually, and physically abused me. It was like hell on earth during that time, and I had always been taught that hell was not a place we wanted to go. I felt deep in my spirit the pit of hell on earth. He hit me, tried to suffocate me, tore off my clothes, and abused me. I was at the lowest point in my life.

I prayed and sought the face of God. I knew if He left me, I would have no one in my life. I held on as tightly as I could to God, but life seemed to be harder than I ever thought it could be. I was in such bondage to Satan and the problems surrounding me that I tried to take my life. It wasn't so much that I wanted to die as I wanted to make the pain from the abuse stop and feel loved.

God helped me through many sorrowful days and nights and brought me through many years. I really had to trust Him with my life. With strength from God, I left the man who abused and tormented me for nineteen months, and I moved on to a better life.

Over the years, physical and mental pain kept increasing. Stress seemed to fill me up in every aspect of work as I tried to make a living for myself and desperately tried to live for God. I knew I shouldn't always be in so much pain, but I didn't know what was wrong. I sought different doctors over the years, but their many diagnoses didn't help—I was told it was just arthritis, back pain, leg pain, headaches, gall bladder problems, or several other diagnoses. Pain does not discriminate. It will attack any age, color or race.

I was raised in the church and saved at age twelve. I came to know the Holy Spirit intimately as I grew up. I had such a desire to know God. I remember writing out books in the Bible just so that I would know it in my heart.

I found joy in the Sword (Bible) drills the church used to have for kids. They would name a verse in the Bible and all the kids would try and find it the fastest and then jump up and read it. God had me on a path to follow Him and it was truly my desire to get close to Him.

Throughout my life, God led me to minister to many people. The Lord gave me a gift of playing the piano and I love playing it. My brother, sister and I would sing a special song in church most every Sunday from the time that I could nearly walk. I used music, and I taught and shared the Word of God on the streets, preaching and praying as I got older. I was a youth pastor for a while and then served as an assistant pastor. I also pastored a church for a few years.

Experiencing so much pain and dealing with the added pressure of being in full-time ministry caused my body to keep going downhill with pain. I would have excruciating pain in my back, legs, feet, and neck. So many things occurred while I was ministering in a full-time capacity, and stressful situations would bombard me with the people within the church. I was dealing with several judgmental, hypocritical people in leaderships positions. Times were tough in the church, and my understanding of God was changing drastically. I had been raised in an evangelical denomination that did not believe in the manifestations of the Holy Spirit in power and speaking in tongues. Clearly, healing and deliverance were not accepted as a plan of God. When I met the charismatic/Pentecostal Christians, I knew that God would work through avenues that I had not seen in the past. God was leading me out of my previous religious understanding and opening my spirit to a "Holy Spirit, have Your way" biblical walk with Him.

I'm so thankful that God opened my eyes to His miracle working power and a deeper, more intimate walk with Him.

Also, I want to add that I believe all that have asked Jesus Christ into their lives, repented of their sins and believe that Jesus died for their sins and rose on the third day from the tomb will have eternal life in heaven with Jesus. It says in John 3:16, *"For God so loved the world that He gave His only begotten Son, that whoever believes in Him should not perish but have everlasting life."*

I don't believe that you have to speak in tongues to make it to heaven, but I do believe that it's a gift from God and a demonstration of His presence in our lives. It says in First Corinthians 14:1, *"Pursue love, and desire spiritual gifts, but especially that you may prophesy. For he who speaks in a tongue does not speak to men but to God, for no one understands him; however, in the spirit he speaks mysteries."* Tongues are a gift from God and we should seek all that God wants to give us.

3

Turn of Events

Before I began full-time ministry, I remarried and had two beautiful children. At this time, I was experiencing pain throughout my body, which seemed to escalate after my second child was born.

I was living in Springfield, Missouri, and had packed the boys—the younger one was only two weeks old—into my compact car for a trip to the store. On my way home, it began to rain. One of the kids distracted me, and before I knew what was happening, I had plowed into the back of a pickup. The car was totaled, crushed to about half its original size. Thank God, the children were not harmed, but I slammed into the steering wheel with my chest on impact.

That was when it seemed my body reached another crossroad of pain, but this was on a completely different, deeper level. I tried to get relief from the tremendous pain any way that I could. There were times when I just couldn't take the pain anymore, and I would cry and get depressed.

I was painting one day and my body started hurting intensely in my back. Next thing I know I was totally unable to move. It took me about four hours to finally crawl to a back seat of a vehicle to go to the hospital. While at the hospital they could not find out any reason why I was in so much pain and sent me home. Pain can do some very bad things to those who are holding on mentally with a thin rope due to their agony. I was reaching out for any help that I could find. I was also getting adjusted by a Chiropractor frequently to see if I could get relief that way as well.

Pain definitely had a strong grip on me. At times, it was so intense I had to pull over in my vehicle to pray and ask God to take it from me. The pain in my back, hips, neck was so excrutiating all I could do was cry. To me it seemed my prayers fell on deaf ears, even though I knew God heard everything I said. But since the doctors had not diagnosed me with Fibromyalgia I was not taking any medications for any pain.

At this time, I really didn't know that a good portion of the pain was due to stress from the situations in which I had been involved and situations from which I needed deliverance, as well as from the food I had eaten over the years.

Our body is a temple of the Holy Spirit. The Old Testament offers an analogy, telling us that the temple represents the outer court (*our body*), inner court (*our soul*), and the Holy of Holies (*our spirit*). Satan seems to attack us in the outer court through afflictions and diseases such as fibromyalgia.

"Do you not know that your body is the temple of the Holy Spirit who is in you, whom you have from God, and you are not your own? For you were bought at a price; therefore glorify God in your body and in your spirit, which are God." (1 Corinthians 6:19-20)

I often offered up prayers, and God would answer, but the pain would still be present in my body. For many years, I couldn't figure out what was going on. The pain would radiate through my neck, down my back, and to my hips, legs, and feet. Even my hands and arms hurt. I would lie in bed at night, tossing and turning, and try to deal with the pain so I could sleep. I had many nights of insomnia and very restless sleep. Hot flashes shot through my body.

I was sick of going to the hospitals and seeing doctors who could not diagnose me with anything but a few minor problems. I was very depressed; life just wasn't what I thought it should be. I was serving God, yet it seemed that life could not get much worse.

Then the ministry itself took a downward spiral, and life in the church was not what I felt God wanted it to be. I reached the point where the pain in my physical body was controlling my spiritual and mental being. I turned my back on the church, and my marriage again fell apart. Pain and depression dictated my life.

I went to the bars to find a little relief in alcohol—if I had enough alcohol in me, then I didn't have to feel the pain anymore—but it was a temporary fix. One thing led to another, and I got on a fast road down the wrong path. For about seven years, I sat on bar stools, conversed with the people of the world with answers to everything but what God wanted, and they would give advice for my problem. I was stuck in a hole of depression and fear. Proverbs 27:19 says, *"As in water face reflects face, So a man's heart reveals the man."* My heart was filled with fear and depression.

One night, I decided to talk to a man named Mark. He had become a friend through the years of sitting on the bar stools. He had previously asked me out and I declined but this night was different and I told him that I would go out with him. We decided to date and then after several months, I felt I wanted to marry him. In the back of my mind, I knew that somehow, things would work out with us. Obviously, I should not have been in a bar to meet a man, but God can work in mysterious ways, especially when people are praying for you. God brought us out of the bar scene; I have not used alcohol to soften the pain since. Mark and I have repented of our sins and have not turned back to them. We haven't drunk alcohol for several years. We had some major issues when we first married, but by God's mercy and grace, we turned our lives over to Him and repeatedly repented. We are walking in the light of His Word and still have our differences but we look to Jesus for His strength. Praise God!

God has led us to minister to others that have backsliden or just haven't given their lives to Him. It's amazing who the Lord puts in our lives and we actually get strength from God as we witness to different people. I'm so thankful that God had mercy on us and His grace covers *all* of our sins.

4

God Gives Hope through Fasting

When the pain was excruciating for very long periods of time, I knew it was time to find out why. I went to three doctors of whom one was a neurological specialist, one was a family doctor (of which I changed since he could not figure out what was wrong), and the other was my new family doctor. The new family doctor and neurologist diagnosed me with hypertension and fibromyalgia. They prescribed blood pressure medication; Lisinopril, and eight different pills for the fibromyalgia, which was Citolapram, Alprazolam, Vitamin D, Zinc, Cyclobenzaprine, Hydrocodone, and a few others that were trial and error type drugs. When I first began taking the medications, it took several months for the doctors to regulate how much to take of each one, since the pain level was so high and it was not under control as of yet.

Pain had a way of dictating my life; it affected how I felt emotionally. My muscles and body hurt so much at times that I didn't want to get out of bed. I was depressed and wondered how I would function in the days ahead, especially if I never felt better. This went on for several years.

Even when I went to the dentist for a tooth extraction my nerves were so shot and messed up, because of the fibromyalgia, that they could not deaden the nerves around the tooth. The tooth I had pulled took thirteen shots to finally get it somewhat numb.

I also went in for a colonoscopy and the anesthesiologist gave me medicine to put me out while they did the procedure and again, due to my nerves that were shot I was awake during the whole procedure and felt the device they put inside of me during the colonoscopy. I should have been out during the whole procedure, but my husband witnessed it and even the doctor could not believe that I was not knocked out. They doubled the dosage of medication to put me out but I was still awake and feeling everything.

All of this time I was trying to allow the doctors to regulate my medications for pain. Mark and I were praying and seeking God with all of our hearts. We were following His desires for our marriage and lives, although we had our days of struggles. We were going to church and making new friends that loved the Lord and trying to be the people that God created us to be. My pain still dictated a lot of our routine. I could barely stand being touched at times, due to the pain. At night, Mark would try to hold me and it would feel as if spiders were crawling on me and every nerve in my body would just go crazy. I couldn't stand having a person touch me when my nerves were so inflamed and irritable.

It was difficult to function as a normal human being, and it weighed heavily on our marriage.

After a couple of years, Mark and I were at church on a Sunday morning. The preacher said he was going to call a twenty-one-day fast for the church people. I definitely wanted to participate, because I knew that fasting breaks the yoke or bondage from our lives. So I began the twenty-one-day "Daniel fast," which required that I eat only fruits and vegetables and drink a lot of water. I did not care for water; it was not something I would drink on a daily, weekly, or even monthly basis. I would have a diet drink first thing in the morning and then drank those throughout the day. Before I went to sleep, if I needed a drink, it would be a diet soda. My first battle arose—trying not to drink a diet soda! Do you know how hard it is to not drink something that you've drunk for years and years? It actually was not as difficult as I thought it would be, but I'm giving all the thanks to God for taking the desire away from me. I have not had one sip of a diet soda to this day. God delivered me from diet soda. I was addicted to it, but when I went through the fast, Jesus broke the yoke!

Even after the fast ended, I continued to eat more healthfully. I ate a lot of fruit, vegetables, Ezekiel bread, nuts, natural butter, natural popcorn, and veggie patties. I didn't eat sugar or meat products. I tried to stay away from milk as much as possible and ate mainly organic foods, frozen and fresh vegetables. The "ribs" and "turkey" patties were made of vegetables. Wheat spaghetti with organic spaghetti sauce was a great source of nourishment. I ate beans and a lot of salads with vinaigrette dressings. I also ate organic peanut butter with no sugar and with blackberries smashed up on top with Ezekiel bread. I made pumpkin bread that was all natural, with no sugar or white flour. I used raw agave nectar as a sweetener. Not everything worked for us—I tasted a soy-milk product but didn't care for it. I thought tofu was good, but my husband really didn't like it—but we did make an effort to change our eating habits.

I cooked without vegetable oil, using only coconut oil and olive oil. The more I ate this way, the better I felt. Before I knew it, the pain had left my body, and I felt like an entirely new person. My blood pressure had dropped to what it was when I was very young—110/78. My energy level was stronger than it had been in years. Of course, my no longer drinking soda and my taking care to eat healthy foods was a big part of it, but God healed me so that I no longer had to take medications on a daily basis. Previously, the level of pain I had when I tried to sleep seemed off the charts. I could barely touch my skin without it hurting. It felt as if there were knots all over my body and in all of my muscles. They would cramp up, spasm, and knot up, and it would make it hard to keep my muscles relaxed and free from tightening and locking up my arms and shoulders.

As I began to eat pineapple, bananas, oranges, strawberries, cantaloupe, kiwi, watermelon, broccoli, cauliflower, green beans, and potatoes—lots of different fruits and vegetables—I felt a change in my body. One day during the fast, I was praying for God to lead me, and I sensed that He was asking me to eat an orange peel. I asked God, "*What? You want me to eat the skin of an orange?*" But I went ahead and ate the peel. Oh yes, it was nasty and bitter, but I ate it anyway. As I was eating it, I kept thinking, *God, I hope you know what you are doing and this isn't poisonous.* After I ate the peel, I decided to go on the Internet and search for information on what an orange peel has in it. I discovered that orange peels contain compounds that have many health benefits, from possibly reducing risk of certain types of cancer to helping to lower cholesterol levels. I ate the orange peel because God had directed me to do so, but I prayed that I wouldn't have to eat it again—regardless of its health benefits. So far, I've had no further direction from the Lord to eat it again. Praise the Lord!

I'm still trying many different foods to see how my body reacts to them, but I do know that white-flour products seem to change my pain levels, and I don't function well after ingesting it. Broccoli and lots of water seems to make me feel very good.

Another culprit that adversely affects me is sugar and sweeteners. I feel much better if I've had water with no sweetener in it. If I do use a sweetener, I use raw stevia, which seem to have no effect on my body.

Caffeine has a bad effect on my being able to cope with fibromyalgia. I had been off all caffeine and sweeteners for a few weeks, and then one day I decided to drink iced tea. I brewed tea and used sweeteners—and that night, I was in tremendous pain and could not sleep. It took a couple of days of drinking lots of water to flush the caffeine and sweeteners out of my body.

Several foods have been trial and error but the end process has been beneficial. A lot of people have different diseases that seem to be lifetime problems, but food may be the cause of the chemical imbalances in the body. Why not try changing your diet just to see if you can get off of medications and be pain free? It's definitely worth the effort!

5

Satan's Plan to Destroy through the Mouth

One of Satan's biggest secrets today is his plan to kill, steal, and destroy God's people, either by corrupting them with sin without repentance or through another avenue—food. The agricultural and food industries have perverted food by using chemicals to cultivate and grow, as well as in food processing. Most people are blind to the diseases and epidemics that these chemicals cause in America.

Salt is in food as a preservative, but most Americans use so much of it at the table and in food preparation that it can lead to elevated blood pressure. I did extensive research on many foods and found that processed foods are power-packed with salt and additives that are destructive to the human body. Everyone needs to check out what they are eating before ingesting it. It's time for America to wake up to the devastating strategies of Satan and the onslaught of diseases that are ruling the lives of many American's. Our water is so filled with chemicals that it should eliminate all the bacteria, but if you could see the bacteria that remain in water, you would not drink it. Many people have switched to bottled water, assuming it's healthier than tap water, but bottled water now seems to be somewhat harmful due to the chemicals that are released into the water from the soft plastic bottles. Others rely on the large water bottles, which don't seem to release the chemicals that the small bottles do. Also, we now have reverse osmosis systems and other filtering systems for water in the home. So the trend to drink from the tap is slowly drifting away unless you have a filtered system to use. Obviously, filtered water is the best that you can drink without all the chemicals that are absorbed through the bottles.

Food and carbonated soda pop seem to contribute to poor health today. What goes in our body feeds the body and can either heal it or destroy it. Again, the thief has come to steal, kill, and destroy each one of us, and what better way than to attack through the use of food and drinks? Food today is so perverted or changed from its natural state that a lot of food is very unhealthy for a person to eat. We live in a fast paced society that wants everything thrown into the microwave and that leads us to processed frozen foods that one can just pop into the electronic wizard. Microwaves are great for a few things, but when we take away the nutrients that are naturally grown in vegetables and fruits then it destroys the nutritional value for our bodies. We live in a fast food restaurant era that's filled with junk food and although, some are changing their menus, there is still a lot of junk food available through these establishments. Intake of refined sugar is harmful to your body. Sugar has been known to be a cancer starting agent. As I've mentioned,

I use raw agave nectar in making different foods. It's a natural, organic sweetener, and it's much healthier for you than refined sugar. Also, coconut oil is very good for those who have inflammation. Inflammation can cause a great deal of pain, fatigue, and restlessness. Inflammation may be due to food intake, stress, or as an indication that something is going on in your body. Inflammation can be deadly, yet we shrug off the problem as if it's just a daily thing that we must live with, popping pills to deal with the pain. We may not take it too seriously, but it is serious! If Satan can get you at a level of pain where you have to take a pill to cope, then he is winning this war on America and the health of Americans. We have cursed ourselves at times by putting destructive garbage in our own mouths. I believe we need a good deal of information on what is healthy and how we can make it benefit the body and live without pain.

When we buy produce at the grocery store, we may throw it in the refrigerator and eat it later—that's a big mistake. We should wash produce with fresh water and scrub it thoroughly, either with fruit and vegetable wash or a drop or so of Dawn dish soap to clean off the chemicals on the outside of potatoes, apples, oranges, and many other vegetables and fruits. A lot of people can't afford to buy organic fruits and vegetables, as these are more expensive than other produce, but they could buy organic dressing, which is comparable in price to other dressings, and is healthy for you.

When I cook spaghetti, I use fresh sauce with fresh vegetables and wheat spaghetti, which is much lighter, without all the starch from regular noodles. If you're a bread eater, the best I have found is the multigrain bread with seven grains. I also eat Ezekiel bread, which is made mainly from vegetables. It's very healthy, but it is more expensive than white bread.

I also eat natural organic peanut butter that has no sugar in it, which tastes very good. Natural garlic and other spices are also healthier for you. Anything fresh is always better. I eat mushrooms, onions, and a lot of greens. Add a little brown rice, and it's a tasty meal. Beans, lettuce, tomatoes, and a corn-based tortilla also make a meal. Fresh salsa is good for you, and multigrain chips are not as unhealthy as regular chips. Always drink water that is filtered, and drink iced tea or coffee without caffeine.

Stretching your muscles even to a small degree will help your body resist the fibromyalgia, nerve issues, inflammation and other problems. Just stretch! It's easy to stand against a door frame and stretch your arms. Satan has linked the comfort of eating destructive foods with tiredness and laziness. If you don't feel up to moving, then look to the one who is trying to kill you through sedentary activities and eating unhealthy foods. If you are a Christian, he wants you to stop living for God, and if you're not a Christian, he wants your entire being. God is faithful and just. He will forgive us our sins, including indulging in food that is for comfort and feels good, as well as our being lazy and not exercising the body that He gave us to take care of for His glory. I was there with most and I indulged for years in pleasurable foods and soda, but God opened my eyes to the dangers of consuming the food of the Enemy and not choosing and cleansing the right food for the temple of the Holy Spirit to dwell in. I'm still working on choosing wisely and am definitely not perfect, but I am striving for what I believe God wants so that I can fulfill what He has called me to do in life—to share the gospel of Jesus Christ with those with whom I come in contact.

God doesn't desire for us to be miserable and live a life of pain and misery. He wants us to be free from the chains of pain, depression, laziness, unbelief, fatigue, and more.

6

The Mind and Mouth Portal

We live in such a perverted society. We can see it on the TV, comparing the shows that we grew up with to the media today. TV is much more perverted than it was forty years ago. If Satan will do it in the media, he will attack the very essence of what is essential for people to survive and live. How much better could Satan have it than to take the very things that we need to live (food and drink) and pervert them to look and taste so enticing—yet eventually these things will kill us? John 10:10 says, *"The thief does not come except to steal, and to kill, and to destroy. I am come that they may have life, and that they may have it more abundantly."*

If this book can help one person to be free from the pain of fibromyalgia, then it will be worth all it took for me to follow the leading of the Holy Spirit to write it. God is a great and wonderful Father, and He wants more than anything for His children to come out of being whipped by Satan and stand up as a child who has been saved by the blood of Jesus—not just for salvation but for healing and deliverance from Satan's plan to destroy God's children.

When Jesus died for our sins, it was to set us free from the works of Satan. Jesus went to the very depths of hell to get the keys of the kingdom of God. Satan has no power over us, God's children, unless we allow him to entice us with food and anything worldly that will hold us in bondage and not serve God at the capacity that He designed. So many Christians are in bondage to something and have not allowed God to free them from the tormenting spirits of darkness that speak to them.

Satan is an angel of light, and although it may seem harmless at times, there are things that we do that bring destruction into our lives, rather than freedom in Christ. I want to be free and not allow pain, depression, fear, doubt, addictions or anything else to hold me in chains of sin. I want to live at the level that God has created for me to live, so that my life will bring glory to the Father through the power of the Holy Spirit.

Daily, I ask God to help me walk with Him and not shrink back into rituals or habits of the past. I want today to be a new day, for the Holy Spirit to lead me, and to be overflowing with the perfect love of God. God loves each of us and wants us to be knowledgeable about how He will heal us. Too many are often just conforming to this world. Jesus said in Romans 12:2, *"And do not be conformed to this world, but be transformed by the renewing of your mind, that you may prove what is that good, and acceptable and perfect will of God."*

How do we get transformed? Read the Word of God and listen to the voice of the Holy Spirit. If you are a child of God, then your spirit is connected to the Holy Spirit. The Holy of Holies, your innermost being that is inside of you, is where Jesus Christ ministers to us through the Holy Spirit. The outer court is where we have the trouble at times—the carnal flesh. We come to God, as they did in the tabernacle in the Old Testament, and pray, but it seems like our prayers are hitting the ceiling and bouncing right back to us. It's because there is a huge battle going on in the outer court.

Remember Zacharias? He had a battle with the angel of the Lord in the outer court of the temple. Because Zacharias couldn't get his confusion under control and believe that God was going to give Elizabeth a child in her old age, God shut his mouth so that what he knew in his heart could not be destroyed through his mouth.

Luke 1:5-22 says, *"There was in the days of Herod, the king of Judea, a certain priest named Zacharias, of the division of Adijah. His wife was of the daughters of Aaron and her name was Elizabeth. And they were both righteous before God, walking in all the commandments and ordinances of the Lord blameless. But they had no child, because Elizabeth was barren, and they were both well advanced in years. So it was, that while he was serving as a priest before God in the order of his division, according to the custom of the priesthood, his lot fell to burn incense when he went into the temple of the Lord. And the whole multitude of the people was praying outside at the hour of incense. Then an angel of the Lord appeared to him standing on the right side of the altar of incense. And when Zacharias saw him, he was troubled, and fear fell upon Him. But the angel said to him, "Do not be afraid, Zacharias, for your prayer is heard, and your wife Elizabeth will bear you a son, and you shall call his name John. And you will have joy and gladness, and many will rejoice at his birth. For he will be great in the sight of the Lord, and shall drink neither wine or strong drink. He will also be filled with the Holy Spirit, even from his mother's womb. And he will turn many of the children of Israel to the Lord their God. He will also go before Him in the spirit and power of Elijah, to turn the hearts of the fathers to the children, and the disobedient to the wisdom of the just, to make ready a people prepared for the Lord. And Zacharias said to the angel, "How shall I know this? For I am an old man and my wife is well advanced in years." And the angel answered and said to him, I am Gabriel, who stands in the presence of God, and was sent to speak to you and bring you these glad tidings. But behold, you will be mute and not able to speak until the day these things take place, because you did not believe my words which will be fulfilled in their own time."*

The tongue is powerful and is used for good or evil. What better place for Satan to sit and entice people than at the mouth portal? The mouth probably is the biggest portal, or access, for Satan to get into a person's life.

Have you ever heard the phrase, "Open mouth; insert foot?" That's because the mouth can be dangerous or unproductive, or it can be used to glorify God. The mouth is powerful. Remember when Adam and Eve were in the Garden of Eden? The mouth was the avenue that Satan used to get to Eve. He tempted her to eat the apple—*eat this, and you will be like God.* He started in the garden and has never stopped enticing people with food. Eve took a bite and then discovered that she was naked, a sinner now in the sight of God. By opening her mouth and having this conversation with Satan, the first couple was kicked out of the Garden of Eden.

If I were Eve, I would have done almost anything to give back the bite of that apple. She probably never wanted to see another apple in her life after that, because it caused so much pain and destruction. They had to till the ground from that point on for food and work. Even if she had seen a tree that had an apple outside of the Garden of Eden, I can't imagine why she would ever eat it—it would be connected to too many memories of how good she had it in the garden. Satan stole the goodness and peace that they had. The innocence, oneness with God, and life in paradise was gone. The perfect life they had lived every day was filled with sin. They'd had a life without stress, spending time with God and taking care of the animals. What a life it must have been—but it all changed with one bite.

My point is this: if Satan started back then in a perfect garden, how much more is he using food today to get to the souls of people? How much more is he using food to get them depressed, in pain, discouraged, and away from God? He's a destroyer of God's children.

7

Pill-Popping Society

Americans seem to live and breathe drugs. They take a drug to breath, a drug to feel better, a drug to make it through the day and to relieve stress, and a drug to calm down. There are drugs for just about anything you want to relieve or change in the body. If you don't want to feel it, there is a pill to numb it.

Pharmakeia is a Greek word used in the Bible that means drugs or sorcery. Strong's Concordance (5331) gives the definition for pharmakeia as:

1. the use or the administering of drugs
2. poisoning
3. sorcery, magical arts, often found in connection with idolatry and fostered by it
4. metaph. the deceptions and seductions of idolatry

The word pharmacy is derived from pharmakeia. Drugs, depending on whether they are legal or illegal, can be used to bless or curse you, but taking drugs is not a simple action. Every time you take drugs, it creates a supernatural response. Drugs don't just affect the body; they affect the biological, physiological, and spiritual part of a person.

My question to you is this: when you take medication, do you pray over it before you take it? Do you ask God to allow the medication to do only what it is intended to do inside of you? Ask the Holy Spirit to bless the medication and not allow Satan to use it for evil against you. Pray, and know that God has allowed this avenue to be the one for your healing. No one wants pain, so we reach for the quick fixes to stop the pain from being excruciating. Migraines, back pain, arthritis, ulcers—no one wants the curse of diseases or pain. But how do we change the direction that America is going with medication? Do we really need medications to change our moods, feelings, chemical imbalances, or pain? Somehow, I think if we could just get to the root of most of these ailments, we would see more deliverance than cures through a pill bottle.

America needs deliverance from stupidity and believing everything they read about cures through multiple pills that may be trial-and-error and cause side effects that create other problems as they attempt to alleviate the current situation. It may sound wonderful when you want to be out of pain, but it's a vicious cycle of death, all to bring people to a place of giving up and not wanting to live, especially for the kingdom of God. God did not leave us to be tormented and in pain. He gave His Son Jesus Christ to bring us out of all the pain and helplessness that was there after sin entered the world.

Most people assume that Jesus came to bring us to a point of salvation, but Jesus said He came to bring us life and to bring it more abundantly. If people are in pain, they don't feel like they are living an abundant lifestyle. An abundant life is a full life; an overflowing, happy life. Jesus knows how to save, deliver, and heal. He's the same yesterday, today, and forever. Stop being caught in allowing foods inside of you that have been prepared to actually destroy your life rather than promote your health. Many people are addicted to junk food and foods that are unhealthy, but just remember God created you to live and not be filled with things that make you feel tired and sick. Christ died on the cross for you, but many are blinded to the truth that He can and will set you free from addictions, from pain and discouragement.

We have to do our part and ask Jesus to come inside of our hearts and clean house. Psalm 34:11-14 says, *"Come, ye children, hearken unto me: I will teach you the fear of the Lord. What man is he that desireth life, and loveth many days, that he may see good? Keep thy tongue from evil, and thy lips from speaking guile. Depart from evil, and do good; Seek peace and pursue it."* Get out of the mind-set of being negative all the time. Life and death are in the power of the tongue. If you speak death, you get death. If you speak life, you get life and have it more abundantly. Stop focusing on the bad in your life. As Christians we should have joy and gladness. See what God has done. If you want to continue bringing curses down on yourself, keep speaking negative things and acknowledging what Satan wants you to dwell on.

Focus on what God is doing in your life and how He is bringing you through every situation, and then watch to see what the Lord will do through you. I hope and pray that you will allow God to open your mouth with food that will heal you and set you free. Psalm 34:8 says, "*Oh taste and see that the Lord is good. Blessed is the man that trusteth in Him.*" *He is faithful and will bring you out of any situation, if you just have faith that He can and will do it. He said that whatever you ask in His name, He will do for you*" (John 14:13).

God loves you and will set you free. Open your heart to the wooing of His Spirit, and He will teach you ways that will bring blessings into your life. God may be asking you to fast to break the yoke of slavery to food, and if so, then just do it. God wants to bless you and keep you until He returns to take His children home. Don't let Satan dupe you out of your blessings. Have faith in God, and He will lead you into all things.

8

Deliverance and Healing for You

Pain is a symptom that likes to take down the whole person. It's not selective in who it attacks, but when it does attack, it tries to gain access not only into the physical part of a person but also the mental and spiritual. Pain that attacks the mind also affects the physical and spiritual part of a person. Anxiety, fear, depression, anger, unforgiveness or whatever grabs hold of a person and creates pain from within is demonstrated in the physical body and in the spiritual being. We seem to question God and His omnipotent power to stop our anxiety, fear, or pain. When a person gets stressed out and takes all the struggles of loneliness, abandonment, or rejection on his or her own shoulders, then the body is attacked in the muscles and nervous system, and it begins to wreak havoc and cause illnesses and diseases, such as fibromyalgia.

Stress is a big factor with fibromyalgia and many other diseases. Until you come to the place of saying, "God, clean out the inward house that You dwell in" and then let Him do it, you will still have the pain and stress, and it will still be attacking your nervous system and your body.

Bitterness, pain, lack of forgiveness, anger, and frustration are all triggers that need to be placed on the throne of God and left there.

If you need to forgive those who have hurt you in the past, then let Jesus be your counselor and tell Him about it. Then let Him heal you from that pain. Forgive those people who offended you or hurt you in the past. It's not worth letting your entire being suffer for things that happened a week ago or fifty years ago. The only way to be free from the chains of pain is to ask Jesus to take away the stress, fear, anxiety, hurt, anger, or lack of forgiveness and to start all over, with your heart filled the power of the Holy Spirit.

Love those who have caused you pain. Forgive them. God can't dwell where there is no forgiveness; where there is bitterness, hatred, anger, malice, envy, or jealousy. He wants to have all of you and not see you suffer from the past. He died on the cross to give us life—not just in heaven but for here on earth as well. You were not created to just suffer on earth; you were created to be a witness of what God has done in your life. How does it look if Christians are always downcast and beaten down with diseases and problems?

God came to set us free from the torment of Satan. God is a restorer through His Son, Jesus. If we give up trying to get all of our ducks in a row and simply lay all of our cares at His feet, then we will have joy unspeakable and peace that transcends all of our understanding. The pain of fibromyalgia is considered a chronic pain—a pain that is ongoing. As a testimony for the Lord Jesus Christ, I can definitely tell you that the pain associated with fibromyalgia is curable through Jesus. I was in so much pain and lived with that pain for years and years. Now, I have been set free from it. I no longer have to take medications to get me through the day so I can function in a somewhat normal manner. Just by listening to the Holy Spirit and changing my diet, as He instructed, the pain dissipated. My God is the healer, deliverer, and restorer of this temple called the body.

Walk in the light of the Holy Spirit. God wants His children free from the lies of the Enemy. Don't settle for less than being a child of the King. God loves you so much that He did the most anyone would ever do to give you hope and healing. God gave His only Son, Jesus Christ, to give you life, hope, and victory in this world. God is love, power, and truth. He extends His mercy and grace to each one of us. There is nothing that God will not forgive you for, if you come to Him with a sincere heart and ask for forgiveness. Even if someone hurt you, just come to Him and ask Jesus to take that lack of forgiveness from you, and then receive His joy and love where that ugliness was inside of you. You are worth everything that God did for you. Please don't hang on to this world's strategies to get even with someone or to get revenge against those who have hurt you. It may be tough, but it will be worth the effort of giving it to Jesus. His blood will cover every sin, if you will just ask Him to take over your pain. Put the pain on the cross and leave it there. There is healing for you!

Let Jesus rise up within you and let those worries be gone. Jesus is always available and waiting on you to let Him have your problems. If you feel the need to pray, say the following:

"Jesus, please forgive me for my stubbornness and holding on to the hurts for so many years. I choose today to lay the pain at Your feet, walk away, and forgive those who have offended me or hurt me. I do not want this pain any longer in my life. I chose to give it all to You. I choose to love those who have hurt me. Thank You, Jesus, for forgiving me and for Your blood that covers all of my sin. Thank You for dying on the cross and rising on the third day.
I believe in a miracle-working God who has been resurrected from the dead. Thank You for having power over death. Thank You that I now have life and can live to the fullest with You. I receive healing in my body; by Your stripes I am healed. I believe You will do what You say and that I am being made whole. Thank You for salvation, healing and deliverance in my life. In Jesus' holy name, Amen."

I hope that you prayed the prayer of faith and will find hope in the things that I've experienced and changed through Jesus Christ.

I am still on my journey towards heaven and am anxiously awaiting the day that I will see my Savior face to face. My dad has also gone on to be with Jesus and I know that he is watching and waiting for all of us to come to heaven as well. I want to see all of my family and friends there too.

Don't wait and put off another day of accepting Him into your life and making Him Lord and Savior. The world will try and lure you into sin and keep you stuck in the past sins, but I can honestly tell you my God is a forgiving God and will forgive you for all of your sins. Blessed is His holy name!

"You are worth everything that God did for you."

"God loves you so much that He did the most anyone would ever do to give you hope and healing."

About the Author

Kathy Vens currently lives in Davenport, Iowa, but grew up in Missouri. She attended Nazarene Bible College and the school of the Holy Spirit, earned the Ellyson Master Teacher award, and has served as a youth pastor, assistant pastor, and pastor. She is an ordained spirit-filled minister and preaches and teaches as God opens the doors for speaking engagements.

CPSIA information can be obtained at www.ICGtesting.com
Printed in the USA
LVOW100530250513

335281LV00001BA/94/P

9 781449 794187